How to Manage your Weight, and be Fitter, Sat on your Arse!

DARREN DAVIES

DEDICATION

To My Mum

CONTENTS

1 INTRODUCTION

Hello. Let's start at the beginning, and let's be honest with ourselves.

You want to lose weight, or you have at least thought about it, but you cannot be bothered to get off your own backside and do something about it. Or, you have tried before and failed, which is not really a good self-advertisement for you to try to do it again!

You must want to do it else you would not have bought this book that you have heard so much about!

Today is the day that you ask yourself these questions:

- Are you happy with the body you are in at the moment?
- Have you let your health get so bad, that it may be the cause of an earlier death?
- Is your current body shape and health the main reason for a possible low self-esteem?
- Does your weight issue have a negative effect on your day's normal routine?
- Are you embarrassed about your visual appearance?

If you have answered honestly, and you do not really like what you have just told yourself, now is the right time to act.

Now is the right time to start afresh, as putting it off and saying you will begin your new healthier lifestyle next week is not good enough, or even fair to yourself. Do you think it is about time you did something for you, and no-one else?

We may have heard of products making exceptional claims such as, "It does exactly what it says on the tin"! Now there is a book that does exactly what is says on the cover.

I, through this book, can help you realize that you can live a healthy lifestyle, and lose inches off your waist, and other unsightly places, in the process.

With the knowledge I will be passing onto you, in this book, you will discover a new, better, 'you'. A 'you' that you have always wanted to be. You will also be wondering why you haven't thought about this yourself.

Well… I am the proof that cutting out foodstuffs containing 'processed' wheat and corn (incl. corn starch), for instance, can have a drastic effect on your waistline.

I, like many others, hate exercise and/or are unable to do so due to physical disabilities. I spend most of my 'life' sat in front of my PC (programming; 3D modeling; surfing; etc.). It's my job, and because my back is not too good, the most exercise I get is walking to the shops.

By just stopping eating fast foods, breads and 'foods that contain corn starch' I have lost a lot of weight. Yes! Sat on my backside in front of my computer and doing minimal exercise, in three weeks, I have lost 10 inches off my waistline. It is amazing. I now longer find it hard to bend over my belly to tie up my shoe-laces or put socks on.

2 FACTS

There are so many 'expensive' dieting courses and fitness regimes out there to choose from, but many of us have not got the funds to pay for them. The only thing we really end up losing is our money, and being disheartened by that we lose interest also.

Today's mass produced foods contain many bloating agents and fillers to make the product more economical to manufacture. All these manufacturers care about is making money, not your waistline. They also want their products to look the most appetizing, and last longer, on the supermarket shelves, and so they place additives and preservatives into the ingredients to help it do so. These additives and preservatives are not 'natural' food sources and cannot be good for us!

Think of it like this:

- *When you make homemade foods from ingredients that you can buy from your local grocers, those separate ingredients could be eaten, in excess, without any harm to our bodies.*

- *But, if you broke down, into separate ingredients, most of today's processed foods and then tried to eat them, also in excess; your body would not be able to digest them. They would also be very hard to swallow.*

It is not about how much or how often we eat, but what we are eating on a daily basis that is the main cause for the growing increases in our population's obesity.

Obesity is not genetic. But if a parent's eating lifestyle is passed down to their children, there is where the problem lies.

Fast food is a convenience, not a way of life.

- *Did you know? Fried foods often take longer to prepare and cook than their steamed, or microwaved, equivalents! The quicker option is healthier and tastes better.*

- *And the washing up is easier too!*

Along with inactivity, overeating is associated with our growing obesity epidemic and a number of diseases. But intelligent eating can improve mood, performance, and energy levels while helping us to stay lean.

In the 1970s, the percentage of the UK population that was classed obese was 2%. We all ate home-cooked meals and only dined out for special occasions. Today, 2012, is has risen to an astonishing 60%, and this is down to the ever increasing trend of eating out at fast food restaurants. Home-cooked meals, from simple ingredients, is now a special occasion.

Again, in the 1970s, the deaths from obese related illnesses and diseases were hardly heard off. In today's world, heart disease, high blood pressure, diabetes and many others are commonly heard about.

It is a genetic trait that we crave sugars and fats, and we will fill up on them for when times when food is not abundant.

Portion sizes have almost doubled since the 1950s. 'Supersize' and 'Value' options, on menus, offer the consumer to opportunity to feel less guilt in buying smaller sizes in multiple orders. But, the only people gaining from this are the sellers. Less, cleverer, packaging lowers overheads for them, and yet we still are charged more and made to think that we are getting more from them.

- *If a treat is had, more, and more often, it stops becoming a treat.*

Studies have shown that inactivity does not contribute to weight gain. It is the poor diet that we are enticed towards by numerous marketing campaigns from the food industry that is the brunt of most of us being overweight.

Shelves are packed with larger packed snacks that are 'made to share', but just how many of those packs are bought with the intent of eating a little now, and finishing the packet later. Then, how many of us hate seeing a packet half finished?

Multi-packs are also leading us down the obese path. We get offered bargains on foods, when the amounts are more than we would really want to buy. This excess is eaten because; they have to be eaten before the next shop, or before the sell-by-date, or just simply because they are there.

Healthy eating is always thought of as boring food. Why does it have to be? Seasoning is your best friend. You could eat the same fish (a cod fillet) every day, and because you seasoned or cooked it differently, and served alternating vegetable add-ons it would be like a totally different meal. The same can be said for the eating of fruit and vegetables too.

I put it to you that it is fast food that is boring, not the healthier choice. A Big Whopper is always the same! Homemade fries decay after a week, but fast-food franchise fries can look the same after a year or more! Surely that cannot be right!

3 SELF-PSYCHOLOGY

There is already negativity in all healthy regimes, just by the bad use of the word: 'LOSE'.

Nobody wants to lose. We all want to win.

How often do you hear people at the local dieting club start their sentences with the words, "This week I have lost…" and "Next week I intend to lose…"

That does sound very self-rewarding, does it?

But how does this sound, "This week I gained two holes on my belt", or "Next week I will be able to get into that dress (or trousers) that I have wanted for ages."

It is not how we 'do' things, that govern whether we enjoy the outcome, but how we approach them. The journey to our goals is the most important part of all. If we do not enjoy that journey we may not finish it, and un-finished, un-enjoyable, journeys are seldom travelled upon again.

Resolutions! Yes, you know the ones we make every year? Most are thought of months before January, but we let them simmer, and often they are forgotten, only to be turned into the following year's resolution.

If you want to give something up, or start something new, is there anything stopping you from doing it at the earliest convenient moment? Let's say, next week. What about now, even?

Act on your 'wants' now. If you wanted an ice-cream, would you put that off until next January? No, I doubt it! You would simply go and get one, straight away, because 'You wanted one'.

Everything looks the same when looked at through frosted glass, if you do not know what is on the other side!

DO NOT DWELL ON THE NEGATIVE.

Suppose that you have a beautiful garden. One plant is not doing so well, so you focus exclusively on that struggling plant. Soon you forget to notice the other beautiful plants.

Likewise, you might dwell on a mistake or shortcoming to the point that you ruin your self-esteem, or even your life. You fail to take into account all the good that exists, all the good that you have done.

When you look into the mirror, do you zero in on what's wrong? Or do you notice what's right—your overall appearance, your smile, and so on? When you find yourself dwelling on what's wrong in yourself or your life, you might think, "Okay, perhaps this is something I can work on. In the meantime, what else is going on? What can I notice that is going well? What would a friend notice in addition to the faults?"

Whereas dwelling on the negative overlooks positives, this distortion actually negates positives. Imagine that someone compliments you for doing a good job. You say, "No big deal." However, it would be much more satisfying to thank the person and think, "I'm really glad that I was able to figure out what was required and do a good job." Then you'd be validating both the giver of the compliment and yourself.

People with self-esteem are not necessarily brighter, more attractive, or more skillful than those who lack self-esteem. The difference really lies in the way we view ourselves. Dwelling on our negative aspects prevents us from enjoying our core worth and what is presently right about ourselves. Thinking "I can't like myself with this or that fault" also blocks self-acceptance, since it makes eliminating our faults a condition   for   worth.

4 EATING TIMES

Before we let loose on the scrumptious recipes, let us first look at what and when we eat:

BREAKFAST:

We are told that this is the most important meal of the day. Who told us that and who told them?

You have awoken from a good night's sleep and during this time your stomach has shrunk, and your spine has expanded due to not carrying your weight. The last thing your stomach needs is to be stuffed with a greasy fry-up.

Instead drink a large glass (approx. 500ml) of non-concentrate fruit juice, with bits (pulp) preferably.

ELEVENSES:

A piece of fruit or even a small 'self-prepared' fruit salad should stop the cravings. Even a healthy-option smoothie would be nice, just to satisfy the appetite. See the Elevenses recipes for ideas.

LUNCH:

Now is the time to fuel up. See the Lunch recipes for ideas.

This will be our main meal for the day. Half of our 'active day' has passed, and we need only need to eat what we need to last us for six hours, or so. This is where is most of our daily calorie intake will be taken.

Meats, Fish and Eggs… Try to avoid the 'fried' option when possible, and instead opt for grilled, boiled, steamed or microwaved! But if you have no choice and have to fry them, use the healthiest oils and use in your pan.

- *If there is still oil in the pan, after the food has been cooked… you have used too much!*

Always try to have at least one of these involved in your lunchtime meal, and compliment them with a variety of vegetables (or fruit!).

Whether you meal is going to be a salad, a soup, seafood, a poultry dish or meat-dish, remember seasoning is your best friend.

Try to avoid sauces of any kind. They taste lovely, but are mainly fats and sugars.

SUPPER (EVENING MEAL):

This is normally the last meal of the day. It is not meant to be the main meal, as most of us have been led to believe.

Evenings are usually relaxing times which do not require as much fuel as the 'active' part of your day.

The average person will spend about four hours, doing hardly any exercise before retiring to bed. Eating a large calorie-laden meal a few hours before sleep is not a good idea. Those calories will only end up being stored as fat in our bodies, as most of them will not get broken down.

The best way to have a final meal of the day would be to have a finale of taste sensations, to satisfy your palette and hunger without taking on an excess of fat-bound calories.

5 RECIPES (SUGGESTIONS)

Elevenses recipes:

Blueberry Cherry Yogurt Smoothie

1 1/2 cups frozen blueberries
3/4 cup frozen cherries
1 banana, peeled
1 cup non-fat plain Greek yogurt
2 drops vanilla essence
1/4 cup water
4 ice cubes

Add the banana, yogurt, stevia, and water into the blender and add the rest of the ingredients. Blend until smooth. Serves 1-2

Strawberry Greek Yogurt Smoothie

1 banana, peeled
10 large fresh strawberries
1 cup non-fat plain Greek yogurt
2 drops berry-flavored essence or sweetener
10-14 ice cubes

Add all of the above ingredients in the blender and blend well.

Basic Berry Smoothie

1 Cup 'Unsweetened' Almond Milk
1 Cup Mixed Fresh or Frozen Berries
1/2 Cup Natural Plain Greek Yogurt
2 Tbsps. Avocado (optional)
Handful of Ice Cubes
1 Tsp. Stevia/Canderel

Chocolate, Peanut Butter and Banana

1 Cup Almond Milk
1 Banana
1 Tbsp. Natural Peanut Butter
1 Tbsp. Natural Cocoa Powder
1 Tsp. Vanilla
1 Tsp. Stevia/Canderel
1 Tsp. Cinnamon
1 Scoop Natural Protein Powder
Handful of Ice Cubes if desired

Protein Frappe

1 Cup Chilled Coffee
1/2 Cup Almond Milk
1 Tsp. Vanilla
1 Tsp. Stevia/Canderel
Handful of Ice Cubes
1 Scoop Protein Powder
Dash of Cinnamon

Banana Oat

1/4 Cup Old-Fashioned Rolled Oats
1/2 Cup Greek Yogurt
1 Tbsp. Agave Nectar
1/4 Tsp. Cinnamon
1/2 Scoop Protein Powder
1 Banana
1/2 Cup Almond Milk

If none of my suggestions appeal to your taste buds, then why not experiment and make your own. A smoothie is broken down into groups:

THE PROTEIN: This is the most important category and should never be missed out. It is the difference between it being a healthy snack or 'treating' yourself. This will keep you full for longer and those blood sugars balanced.

Always buy plain protein powder and add your own flavor! You want Chocolate? Nothing easier or better tasting than just adding natural cocoa powder and some Stevia/Canderel to any Smoothie Protein you choose. Yummy Chocolate without the added sugar or chemicals!

Same with your yogurt! They say "low-fat strawberry" but most are loaded with chemicals and/or sugar. Natural is always your best choice.

Greek Natural, Plain Yogurt
Natural, Plain Whey Protein Powder
Natural, Plain Yogurt
Natural, Soy Protein Powder
Tofu
Natural, Plain Brown Rice Protein
Natural, Plain Hemp Protein

THE LIQUID: Always add water for consistency. When using 'milks', go for half milk-to-water.

Almond Milk
Brewed, chilled Chai Tea
Coconut Milk
Coffee
Green Tea
Rice milk
Skim Milk
Soy Milk

THE FLAVOUR: There are so many ways to make your shakes to die for. Here are a few:

Almond Extract
Canned Pumpkin
Chai Tea
Cinnamon
Coffee
Ginger
Green Tea
Mint leafs or Extract
Natural Coco Powder
Natural Peanut Butter
Pumpkin Pie Spice
Pure, Vanilla Extract

THE FRUIT AND NUTS: Having frozen fruit on hand makes these smoothies thick and cold. Cutting up bananas before you freeze them makes the blending process that much easier.

Banana
Blackberries
Blueberries
Cherries
Dates
Dried fruits (Currants; Sultanas; etc.)
Fig
Kiwi
Mango
Melon
Orange (or any Citrus alternative)
Papaya
Peach
Pineapple
Pumpkin
Raspberries
Rhubarb
Strawberries

Almond
Cashew
Hazelnut
Peanut
Pecan
Walnut

As you can see the combinations are almost endless. Unleash that creative flair!

Lunch recipes:

'Dug's Easy Omelet':

First, have your filling prepared and ready to hand. Vegetables should be sautéed. Cheese should be pre-sliced or grated. If using left-overs, pre-heat them in a microwave before adding them.

If your omelet pan is not non-stick, spray it with cooking spray before placing it over a medium heat. While the pan is heating, beat two eggs in a bowl with a fork. Do not add milk or any water to the mix.

Add a little oil, or non-salted butter, into your hot pan and make sure the bottom is completely covered. Then pour in your beaten egg mix all at once. When the bottom of the egg has set, lift the edges with a spatula and tip the pan to let the raw mix flow underneath it. Repeat until there is no 'runny' mix left.

Turn down the heat to the lowest setting. If using an electric hob, remove the pan from the heat until the rings cool down.

Place your filling(s) on one half on the omelet only. Continue cooking for a further two minutes or until the egg becomes non-translucent (not shiny).

Once done, flip the un-filled side of the omelet on top of the other and then slide it onto a plate, season and serve.

Mexican Omelet

1 tablespoon (14g) non-salted butter
2 eggs, beaten
2 ounces (55g) jalapeño Jack cheese, shredded or sliced
2 tablespoons (32g) salsa

Make your omelet according to Dug's Easy Omelet, placing the cheese over half of your omelet when you're ready to add the filling.

Cover; turn the heat to low, and cook until the cheese is melted (3 to 4 minutes). Follow the directions to finish making the omelet. Top with salsa and hot

Yield: 1 serving: 5g of carbohydrates; 1g fiber; 4g usable carbs; 25g protein.

Club Omelet

2 slices bacon, cooked and drained
2 ounces (55g) turkey/chicken breast slices
½ small tomato, sliced
1 scallion/gibbon/shallot/spring onion, sliced
2 eggs
1 tablespoon (15g) low-fat mayonnaise

Have your bacon cooked and drained—I like to microwave mine and crumble it up. Cut the chicken/turkey into small squares and have the tomato and scallion sliced and at hand.

Beat the eggs, and make your omelet according to Dug's Easy Omelet, adding just the bacon and poultry while it's still cooking.

Once it's cooked to your liking, sprinkle the tomato and scallion over the meat, spread the mayo on the other side, fold, and serve.

Yield: 1 serving: 29g protein; 5g carbohydrate; 1g dietary fiber; 4g usable carbs.

Crab/Tuna Omelet

¼ cup (35g) canned crab/tuna meat, flaked and picked over for shells and cartilage
2 scallions, sliced, including the crisp part of the green
1 tablespoon (14g) unsalted butter
2 eggs, beaten
1 to 2 tablespoons (14g) low-fat mayonnaise

Mix the meat with the scallions and have the mixture standing by. Make your omelet according to Dug's Easy Omelet, spreading mayonnaise over half the omelet and topping it with the mixture when you're ready to add the filling.

Yield: 1 serving: 3g carbohydrates; 1g fiber; 2g usable carbs; 19g protein.

'The Fridge' Omelet

½ red bell pepper, cut into thin strips
¼ medium onion, thinly sliced
3 tablespoons (45ml) olive oil
2 eggs, beaten
1 ounce (30g) jalapeño jack, shredded or sliced
½ black avocado, sliced

In your pan over medium-high heat, sauté the pepper and onion in the oil until the onion is translucent and the pepper is going limp. Remove from the pan, drain away any excess oil, and keep on hand.

Make your omelet according to Dug's Easy Omelet. Put the cheese on half the omelet and top with the avocado and then the pepper and onion. Cover, turn the heat to low, and let it cook until the cheese is melted. Fold and serve.

Yield: 1 serving: 14g carbohydrates; 6g fiber; 8g usable carbs; 21g protein. (This also contains a whopping 821 milligrams of potassium!)

Greek Salad

1 large head romaine lettuce
1 cup (60g) chopped fresh parsley ½ cucumber, sliced
1 green pepper, sliced
Greek Lemon Dressing
¼ sweet red onion, thinly sliced into rings
12 Greek olives
2 ripe tomatoes, cut into wedges
4ounces (115g) feta cheese, crumbled
Anchovy fillets packed in olive oil (if desired)

Wash and dry your romaine and break or cut it into bite-sized pieces. Cut up and add the parsley, cucumber, and green pepper. (You can do this step ahead of time, if you like, which makes this salad very doable on a weeknight.)

Just before serving, pour on the Greek dressing and toss the salad like crazy.

Arrange the onions, olives, and tomatoes artistically on top and sprinkle the crumbled feta in the middle. You can also add the anchovies at this point, if you know that everybody likes them, but I prefer to make them available for those who like them to put on their individual serving.

Yield: 4 servings: 16g carbohydrates; 6g fiber; 10g usable carbs; 11g protein.

Autumn Salad

2 tablespoons (28g) unsalted butter
½ cup (60g) chopped walnuts
10 cups (200g) loosely packed assorted greens (romaine, red leaf lettuce, and fresh spinach)
¼ sweet red onion, thinly sliced
¼ cup (60ml) olive oil
2 teaspoons wine vinegar
2 teaspoons lemon juice
¼ teaspoon spicy brown or Dijon mustard
pinch of salt
pinch of pepper
½ ripe pear, chopped
1/3 cup (40g) crumbled blue cheese

Melt the butter in a small, heavy saucepan over medium heat. Add the walnuts and let them toast in the butter, stirring occasionally, for about 5 minutes.

While the walnuts are toasting (and make sure you keep an eye on them and don't burn them) wash and dry your greens and put them in salad bowl with the onion. Toss in the oil first. Then combine the vinegar, lemon juice, mustard, salt, and pepper and add that to the salad bowl. Toss until everything is well covered.

Top the salad with the pear, the warm toasted walnuts, and the crumbled blue cheese. Serve.

Yield: 4 generous servings: 13g carbohydrates; 6g fiber; 7g usable carbs; 10g protein.

Greek Lemon Dressing

The use of lemon juice in place of vinegar in salad dressings is distinctively Greek.

¾ cup (180 ml) extra-virgin olive oil
¼ cup (60 ml) lemon juice
2 tablespoons (10.8 g) dried oregano, crushed
1 clove garlic, crushed
Salt and pepper

Put all the ingredients in a container with a tight-fitting lid and shake well.

Yield: 12 servings: 1g carbohydrates; trace of fiber; trace of protein.

This is best made at least a few hours in advance, but don't try to double the recipe and keep it around. Lemon juice just doesn't hold its freshness the way vinegar does.

Blue Cheese Dressing

2 cups (450g) low-fat mayonnaise
½ cup (120ml) buttermilk
½ cup (115g) small-curd cottage cheese
½ teaspoon Worcestershire sauce
1 clove garlic, crushed
1 teaspoon salt
3 ounces (85g) crumbled blue cheese

Whisk together the mayonnaise, buttermilk, cottage cheese, Worcestershire, garlic, and salt, mixing well. Gently stir in the blue cheese to preserve some chunks. Store in a container with a tight-fitting lid.

Yield: Makes roughly 3 cups (720ml): A 2-tablespoon (30ml) serving has 1g carbohydrates; trace of fiber; 2g protein.

California Soup

1 large or 2 small, very ripe black avocados, pitted, peeled, and cut into chunks

1 quart (960ml) chicken broth, heated

Put the avocados in a blender with the broth, purée until very smooth, and serve.

Yield: 2 servings (hot or cold): 6g carbohydrates; 2g fiber; 4g usable carbs; 8g protein.

If you like curry, you've got to try this: Melt a tablespoon (14g) or so of unsalted butter in a small saucepan and add ½ teaspoon or so of curry powder. Cook for just a minute and then add the mixture to the blender with the broth and avocados.

Broccoli Blue Cheese Soup

I'd never had soup made with blue cheese before, but this is amazing.

1 cup (160g) chopped onion
2 tablespoons (28g) unsalted butter
1 turnip, peeled and diced
1½ quarts (1.4L) chicken broth
1 pound (455g) frozen broccoli, thawed
1 cup (240ml) coconut milk
¼ cup (60ml) heavy cream
1 cup (120g) crumbled blue cheese

In a large saucepan, sauté the onion in the butter over medium-low heat (you don't want it to brown).

When the onion's soft and translucent, add the turnip and the chicken broth to the pot. Bring the mixture to a simmer and let it simmer over medium-low heat for 20 to 30 minutes.

Add the thawed broccoli and let it simmer for another 20 minutes.

Scoop the vegetables out with a slotted spoon and place them in a blender. Add a ladleful of the broth and run the blender until the vegetables are finely puréed. Return the mixture to the pot.

Stir in the coconut milk, the heavy cream, and the blue cheese. Simmer for another 5 to 10 minutes, stirring occasionally, and serve.

Yield: 3 servings: 28g protein; 18g carbohydrate; 6g dietary fiber; 12g usable carbs.

'Simply Microwaved' Fish

Not only is this simple, but it's lightning-quick, too.

1 fillet (about 170g) mild white fish
1 tablespoon (14g) unsalted butter
1 tablespoon (3.8g) minced fresh parsley
Wedge of lemon

Place the fish onto a plate and lightly butter it on the top side. Place into a microwave for 2 to 3 minutes. Remove and sprinkle with half the parsley. Turn it over with a spatula before returning it to the microwave for a further 2 minutes, or until the fish is opaque and flakes easily.

Transfer to serving plates, top with the remaining minced parsley, and serve with a wedge of lemon.

Yield: 1 serving: Trace of carbohydrates; no fiber; 31g protein.

Chinese Steamed Fish

12 ounces (340g) cod fish fillets
2 tablespoons (30ml) dry sherry
1 tablespoon (15ml) soy sauce
2 teaspoons grated ginger
½ teaspoon minced garlic or 1 clove garlic, crushed
1½ teaspoons toasted sesame oil
1 or 2 scallions, minced (optional)

Lay the fish fillets on a piece of heavy-duty aluminum foil and turn the edges of the foil up to form a lip.

Mix together the sherry, soy sauce, ginger, garlic, and sesame oil.

If you have not got a steamer, fit a rack (a cake-cooling rack works nicely) into a large casserole dish. Pour about ¼ inch (6mm) of water in the bottom of the skillet and turn the heat to high.

Place the foil with the fish on it on the rack. Carefully pour the sherry mixture over the fish. Cover the pan tightly.

Cook for 5 to 7 minutes or until the fish flakes easily. Serve with minced scallions as a garnish, if desired.

Yield: 2 servings: 2g carbohydrates; no fiber; 31g protein.

Each serving has only 195 calories!

Thai Chicken Bowls

8 boneless, skinless, boneless chicken thighs, cubed (a little over 2¼lbs/1 kg)
2 cloves garlic, crushed
½ cup (80g) chopped onion
2 stalks celery, sliced
2 teaspoons grated ginger
1 teaspoon five-spice powder
½ teaspoon salt
1 tablespoon (15ml) lemon juice
1 teaspoon hot pepper sauce (optional)
28 ounces (850 ml) chicken broth
1 head cauliflower
Guar or xanthan
6 tablespoons (35g) sliced scallions
6 tablespoons (24g) chopped cilantro

Place the chicken in a slow cooker. Top with the garlic, onion, celery, ginger, five-spice powder, salt, and lemon juice.

In a bowl, combine the hot pepper sauce, if using, with the broth and pour it into the slow cooker. Cover the slow cooker, set it to low, and let it cook for 5 to 6 hours.

Run the cauliflower through the shredding blade of your food processor to make cauli-rice. Put the cauli-rice in a microwaveable casserole dish with a lid, add a couple of tablespoons (30ml) of water, cover, and microwave on high for 6 minutes.

Thicken up the sauce in the slow cooker with a little guar or xanthan to about the texture of heavy cream.

Okay, the cauli-rice is done! Uncover it immediately, drain, and divide it into 6 bowls. Divide the chicken mixture, ladling it over the cauli-rice. Top with the scallions and cilantro.

Yield: 6 servings: Each with 20g protein; 4g carbohydrate; 1g dietary fiber; 3g usable carbs.

French Country Chicken with Root Vegetables, Cabbage, and Herbs

5 pounds (2.3kg) skinned chicken breast
1½ tablespoons (23ml) olive oil
1½ tablespoons (21g) butter
2 medium turnips, cut into ½-inch (1.3-cm) cubes
2 medium carrots, cut into ½-inch (1.3-cm) slices
1 medium onion, cut into ¼-inch (6mm) half-rounds
1 head cabbage
4 cloves garlic, crushed
½ teaspoon dried rosemary
½ teaspoon dried thyme
½ teaspoon dried basil
2 bay leaves, crumbled

In a big, heavy saucepan, brown the chicken on both sides in the oil and butter over medium-high heat.

When the chicken is browned all over, remove it to a plate and reserve. Some extra fat will have accumulated in the skillet. Pour off all but a couple of tablespoons (30ml) and then add the turnips, carrots, and onion. Sauté those, scraping the tasty brown bits off the bottom of the pan as you stir, until they're getting a touch of gold, too.

Transfer the sautéed vegetables to a slow cooker.

Cut the cabbage into eighths and put it on top of the vegetables. Arrange the chicken on top of the cabbage. Sprinkle the garlic over the chicken and vegetables. Make sure some ends up on the chicken and some down among the vegetables. Sprinkle the rosemary, thyme, basil, and bay leaves into the slow cooker, making sure some gets down into the vegetables. Season with salt and pepper. Cover the slow cooker, set it to low, and let it cook for 6 to 7 hours.

Yield: 8 servings: Each with 36g protein; 6g carbohydrate; 2g dietary fiber; 4g usable carbs.

Beef Stroganoff

1 pound (455g) ground beef
1 medium onion, diced
1 clove garlic, crushed
1 can 115g) mushrooms, drained
1 teaspoon liquid beef broth concentrate
2 tablespoons (30ml) Worcestershire sauce
1 teaspoon paprika
¾ cup (180g) sour cream
Salt and pepper to taste

Brown and crumble the ground beef in a heavy saucepan over medium heat. Add the onion and garlic as soon as there's a little grease in the bottom of the pan and cook until all pinkness is gone from the ground beef.

Drain the excess grease. Add the mushrooms, broth concentrate, Worcestershire, and paprika. Stir in the sour cream and then add salt and pepper to taste. Heat through, but don't let it boil. This is great as-is, but you may certainly serve it over egg-noodles for the non-low-carb set.

Yield: 3 servings: Each with 9g carbohydrates; 2g fiber; 7g usable carbs; 28g protein.

Southwestern Stuffed Peppers

This was one of those recipes you just come up with out of what's in the house at the time.

1 pound (455g) ground beef
½ cup (80g) chopped onion
1 clove garlic, crushed
1 can (410g) tomatoes with green chilies, divided
1 egg
½ cup (120ml) half-and-half
½ cup (70g) pork rind crumbs
1 teaspoon ground cumin
1 teaspoon salt
½ teaspoon pepper
3 big, nicely shaped green peppers

Preheat oven to 350°F (180°C, or gas mark 4)

In a large bowl combine the ground beef, onion and garlic, ½ cup (120g) of the tomatoes with chilies, the egg, half-and-half, pork rind crumbs, and seasonings.

Use clean hands to combine everything well.

Cut the peppers in half from top to bottom and scoop out the seeds and core. Form the meat mixture into 6 equal balls and press each into a pepper half, mashing it down a little to fill the peppers. Arrange peppers in a baking pan as you stuff them.

Spoon the remaining tomatoes over the top and bake for 75 to 90 minutes.

Yield: This makes 6 servings from 1lb (455g) of ground beef, which is pretty impressive! It's filling, too.

Each serving has 9g carbohydrate; 2g fiber; a usable carb total of 7g; 27g protein.

Lemon-Ginger Pork Chops

1 pound (455g) pork chops, 1 inch (2.5 cm) thick
1 tablespoon (6g) grated ginger
1 tablespoon (15ml) olive oil
1 tablespoon (15ml) soy sauce
1 tablespoon (15ml) dry sherry
1½ teaspoons lemon juice
1 tablespoon (15ml) water
½ clove garlic, crushed
¼ teaspoon toasted sesame oil
¼ teaspoon Stevia/Canderel
1 scallion, sliced, including the crisp part of the green shoot

In a large, heavy saucepan over medium-high heat, brown the pork chops on both sides in the olive oil. Mix together everything else but the scallion and pour into the pan. Turn the chops to coat both sides. Cover the pan, turn the heat to low, and let the chops simmer for 30 to 40 minutes. Spoon pan juices over chops and top with a little sliced scallion to serve.

Yield: 3 servings: Each will have 24g protein; 1g carbohydrate; trace dietary fiber; 1g usable carb.

Pork Slow Cooker Chili

2½ pounds (1.1kg) boneless pork loin, cut into 1-inch (2.5-cm) cubes
1 tablespoon (15ml) olive oil
1 can (410g) tomatoes with green chilies
¼ cup (40g) chopped onion
¼ cup (30g) diced green bell pepper
1 clove garlic, crushed
1 tablespoon (7.8g) chili powder

In a big, heavy saucepan, heat the oil and brown the pork all over. Transfer the pork to a slow cooker. Stir in the tomatoes, onion, pepper, garlic, and chili powder. Cover the slow cooker, set it to low, and let it cook for 6 to 8 hours.

Serve this with sour cream and crumbled Blue cheese, if you like, but it's darned good as-is.

Yield: 8 servings: Each with 25g protein; 3g carbohydrate; 1g dietary fiber; 2g usable carbs.

Supper recipes (there are none):

Whether you call it dinner or supper, this mealtime is normally the last main food intake of the day, and should not be heavy of your stomach. Noodles, salads, seafood, casseroles/stews or light curries are what we should be looking at here.

The last thing we want before we go to sleep is huge meal filled with oil, carbs or calories.

Pick one of the recipe suggestions, for the other meals of the day, and be a little adventurous.

If you do not feel hungry, do not eat but have a cold soup instead.

6 SUMMARY AND FINAL THOUGHTS

Remember, this is not a diet. It is a new way treating of your body better. The word 'diet' instantly brings thoughts of 'going without', hardship, regimental calorie watching, constantly weighing, etc.

Stop calling your new lifestyle a 'diet' and it will not seem harsh at all. Enjoy it. Enter your new life will a positive outlook and reap the rewards.

This way of healthy eating will probably lead to a better night's sleep, as fidgeting and tossing-and-turning in bed is often a sign of your body trying to burn off those excess calories. And, a better sleeping pattern strengthens our own feelings of self-wellbeing, as there is one less thing to worry about.

There are no truer words than these; "You are what you eat".

One final thought… Drink water often.

Most off the bad stuff in the foods that we eat every day without knowing; can be flushed out of our system. If we do not flush them out, they must be going somewhere!